Positive things about today:

_____
_____
_____
_____
_____

What could have made the day better?

_____
_____
_____
_____
_____

How can you better deal with difficulties in the future?

_____
_____
_____
_____
_____

What can you be grateful for today?

_____
_____
_____
_____

Rate the Day

★ ★ ★ ★ ★

Date: / / M T W T F S S

Hours of Sleep: _____

Today's Mood

Morning: Afternoon: Evening:

_____   _____   _____

_____   _____   _____

_____   _____   _____

Did you feel any of the following today?

- [ ] Sad
- [ ] Hopeless
- [ ] Nervous
- [ ] Angry / Frustrated
- [ ] Low Energy / Fatigue
- [ ] Difficulty Concentrating
- [ ] Increase or Decrease in Appetite
- [ ] Other: _____

Food & Beverages

B: _____

L: _____

D: _____

Other: _____

Water

- [ ] [ ] [ ] [ ] [ ] [ ] [ ] [ ]

What impacted your mood today?

_____

_____

_____

_____

_____

_____

Positive things about today:

_____
_____
_____
_____
_____

What could have made the day better?

_____
_____
_____
_____

How can you better deal with difficulties in the future?

_____
_____
_____
_____

What can you be grateful for today?

_____
_____
_____
_____

Rate the Day

★ ★ ★ ★ ★

Date: / / M T W T F S S

Hours of Sleep: _____

Today's Mood

Morning: Afternoon: Evening:

_____   _____   _____

_____   _____   _____

_____   _____   _____

Did you feel any of the following today?

- [ ] Sad
- [ ] Hopeless
- [ ] Nervous
- [ ] Angry / Frustrated
- [ ] Low Energy / Fatigue
- [ ] Difficulty Concentrating
- [ ] Increase or Decrease in Appetite
- [ ] Other: _____

Food & Beverages

B: _____

L: _____

D: _____

Other: _____

Water

- [ ] [ ] [ ] [ ] [ ] [ ] [ ] [ ]

What impacted your mood today?

_____

_____

_____

_____

_____

_____

Positive things about today:

_____
_____
_____
_____
_____

What could have made the day better?

_____
_____
_____
_____

How can you better deal with difficulties in the future?

_____
_____
_____
_____

What can you be grateful for today?

_____
_____
_____
_____

Rate the Day

★ ★ ★ ★ ★

Date: /   /   M T W T F S S

Hours of Sleep: _____

Today's Mood

Morning: _____ Afternoon: _____ Evening: _____

_____ _____ _____

_____ _____ _____

Did you feel any of the following today?

- ☐ Sad
- ☐ Hopeless
- ☐ Nervous
- ☐ Angry / Frustrated
- ☐ Low Energy / Fatigue
- ☐ Difficulty Concentrating
- ☐ Increase or Decrease in Appetite
- ☐ Other: _____

Food & Beverages

B: _____

L: _____

D: _____

Other: _____

Water

☐ ☐ ☐ ☐ ☐ ☐ ☐ ☐

What impacted your mood today?

_____

_____

_____

_____

_____

_____

Positive things about today:

_____
_____
_____
_____
_____

What could have made the day better?

_____
_____
_____
_____
_____

How can you better deal with difficulties in the future?

_____
_____
_____
_____
_____

What can you be grateful for today?

_____
_____
_____
_____
_____

Rate the Day

★ ★ ★ ★ ★

Date: / / M T W T F S S

Hours of Sleep: _____

Today's Mood

Morning: Afternoon: Evening:

_____   _____   _____

_____   _____   _____

_____   _____   _____

Did you feel any of the following today?

☐ Sad

☐ Hopeless

☐ Nervous

☐ Angry / Frustrated

☐ Low Energy / Fatigue

☐ Difficulty Concentrating

☐ Increase or Decrease in Appetite

☐ Other: _____

Food & Beverages

B: _____

L: _____

D: _____

Other: _____

Water

☐ ☐ ☐ ☐ ☐ ☐ ☐ ☐

What impacted your mood today?

_____

_____

_____

_____

_____

_____

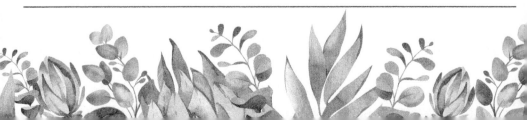

Positive things about today:

_____
_____
_____
_____
_____

What could have made the day better?

_____
_____
_____
_____

How can you better deal with difficulties in the future?

_____
_____
_____
_____

What can you be grateful for today?

_____
_____
_____
_____

Rate the Day

★ ★ ★ ★ ★

Date: /   /   M T W T F S S

Hours of Sleep: _____

Today's Mood

Morning: _____   Afternoon: _____   Evening: _____

_____   _____   _____

_____   _____   _____

Did you feel any of the following today?

- [ ] Sad
- [ ] Hopeless
- [ ] Nervous
- [ ] Angry / Frustrated
- [ ] Low Energy / Fatigue
- [ ] Difficulty Concentrating
- [ ] Increase or Decrease in Appetite
- [ ] Other: _____

Food & Beverages

B: _____

L: _____

D: _____

Other: _____

Water

- [ ] [ ] [ ] [ ] [ ] [ ] [ ] [ ]

What impacted your mood today?

_____

_____

_____

_____

_____

_____

Positive things about today:

_____
_____
_____
_____
_____

What could have made the day better?

_____
_____
_____
_____

How can you better deal with difficulties in the future?

_____
_____
_____
_____

What can you be grateful for today?

_____
_____
_____
_____

Rate the Day

★ ★ ★ ★ ★

Date: / / M T W T F S S

Hours of Sleep: _____

Today's Mood

Morning: _____ Afternoon: _____ Evening: _____

_____ _____ _____

_____ _____ _____

Did you feel any of the following today?

- [ ] Sad
- [ ] Hopeless
- [ ] Nervous
- [ ] Angry / Frustrated
- [ ] Low Energy / Fatigue
- [ ] Difficulty Concentrating
- [ ] Increase or Decrease in Appetite
- [ ] Other: _____

Food & Beverages

B: _____

L: _____

D: _____

Other: _____

Water

- [ ] [ ] [ ] [ ] [ ] [ ] [ ] [ ]

What impacted your mood today?

_____

_____

_____

_____

_____

_____

Positive things about today:

_____
_____
_____
_____
_____

What could have made the day better?

_____
_____
_____
_____

How can you better deal with difficulties in the future?

_____
_____
_____
_____

What can you be grateful for today?

_____
_____
_____
_____

Rate the Day

★ ★ ★ ★ ★

Date: / /   M T W T F S S

Hours of Sleep: _____

Today's Mood

Morning: Afternoon: Evening:

_____   _____   _____

_____   _____   _____

_____   _____   _____

Did you feel any of the following today?

☐ Sad

☐ Hopeless

☐ Nervous

☐ Angry / Frustrated

☐ Low Energy / Fatigue

☐ Difficulty Concentrating

☐ Increase or Decrease in Appetite

☐ Other: _____

Food & Beverages

B: _____

L: _____

D: _____

Other: _____

Water

☐ ☐ ☐ ☐ ☐ ☐ ☐ ☐

What impacted your mood today?

_____

_____

_____

_____

_____

_____

Positive things about today:

_____
_____
_____
_____
_____

What could have made the day better?

_____
_____
_____
_____
_____

How can you better deal with difficulties in the future?

_____
_____
_____
_____
_____

What can you be grateful for today?

_____
_____
_____
_____
_____

Rate the Day

★ ★ ★ ★ ★

Date: ___ / ___ / ___   M T W T F S S

Hours of Sleep: _____

Today's Mood

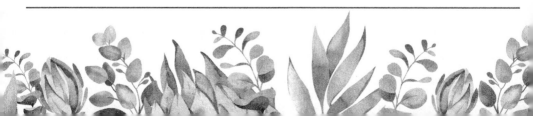

Morning: Afternoon: Evening:

_____   _____   _____

_____   _____   _____

_____   _____   _____

Did you feel any of the following today?

☐ Sad

☐ Hopeless

☐ Nervous

☐ Angry / Frustrated

☐ Low Energy / Fatigue

☐ Difficulty Concentrating

☐ Increase or Decrease in Appetite

☐ Other: _____

Food & Beverages

B: _____

L: _____

D: _____

Other: _____

Water

☐ ☐ ☐ ☐ ☐ ☐ ☐ ☐

What impacted your mood today?

_____

_____

_____

_____

_____

_____

Positive things about today:

_____
_____
_____
_____
_____

What could have made the day better?

_____
_____
_____
_____

How can you better deal with difficulties in the future?

_____
_____
_____
_____

What can you be grateful for today?

_____
_____
_____
_____

Rate the Day

★ ★ ★ ★ ★

Date: / / M T W T F S S

Hours of Sleep: _____

Today's Mood

Morning: _____ Afternoon: _____ Evening: _____

_____ _____ _____

_____ _____ _____

Did you feel any of the following today?

☐ Sad

☐ Hopeless

☐ Nervous

☐ Angry / Frustrated

☐ Low Energy / Fatigue

☐ Difficulty Concentrating

☐ Increase or Decrease in Appetite

☐ Other: _____

Food & Beverages

B: _____

L: _____

D: _____

Other: _____

Water

☐ ☐ ☐ ☐ ☐ ☐ ☐ ☐

What impacted your mood today?

_____

_____

_____

_____

_____

_____

Positive things about today:

_____
_____
_____
_____
_____

What could have made the day better?

_____
_____
_____
_____
_____

How can you better deal with difficulties in the future?

_____
_____
_____
_____
_____

What can you be grateful for today?

_____
_____
_____
_____
_____

Rate the Day

★ ★ ★ ★ ★

Date: / / M T W T F S S

Hours of Sleep: _____

Today's Mood

Morning: _____

Afternoon: _____

Evening: _____

Did you feel any of the following today?

- ☐ Sad
- ☐ Hopeless
- ☐ Nervous
- ☐ Angry / Frustrated
- ☐ Low Energy / Fatigue
- ☐ Difficulty Concentrating
- ☐ Increase or Decrease in Appetite
- ☐ Other: _____

Food & Beverages

B: _____

L: _____

D: _____

Other: _____

Water

☐ ☐ ☐ ☐ ☐ ☐ ☐ ☐

What impacted your mood today?

_____
_____
_____
_____
_____
_____

Positive things about today:

_____
_____
_____
_____
_____

What could have made the day better?

_____
_____
_____
_____

How can you better deal with difficulties in the future?

_____
_____
_____
_____

What can you be grateful for today?

_____
_____
_____
_____

Rate the Day

★ ★ ★ ★ ★

Date: / /   M T W T F S S

Hours of Sleep: _____

Today's Mood

Morning:	Afternoon:	Evening:
_____	_____	_____
_____	_____	_____
_____	_____	_____

Did you feel any of the following today?

☐ Sad

☐ Hopeless

☐ Nervous

☐ Angry / Frustrated

☐ Low Energy / Fatigue

☐ Difficulty Concentrating

☐ Increase or Decrease in Appetite

☐ Other: _____

Food & Beverages

B: _____

L: _____

D: _____

Other: _____

Water

☐ ☐ ☐ ☐ ☐ ☐ ☐ ☐

What impacted your mood today?

_____
_____
_____
_____
_____
_____

Positive things about today:

_____

_____

_____

_____

_____

What could have made the day better?

_____

_____

_____

_____

_____

How can you better deal with difficulties in the future?

_____

_____

_____

_____

_____

What can you be grateful for today?

_____

_____

_____

_____

_____

Rate the Day

★ ★ ★ ★ ★

Date: / /   M T W T F S S

Hours of Sleep: _____

Today's Mood

Morning: _____

Afternoon: _____

Evening: _____

_____

_____

_____

Did you feel any of the following today?

☐ Sad
☐ Hopeless
☐ Nervous
☐ Angry / Frustrated
☐ Low Energy / Fatigue
☐ Difficulty Concentrating
☐ Increase or Decrease in Appetite
☐ Other: _____

Food & Beverages

B: _____

L: _____

D: _____

Other: _____

Water

☐ ☐ ☐ ☐ ☐ ☐ ☐ ☐

What impacted your mood today?

_____

_____

_____

_____

_____

_____

Positive things about today:

_____
_____
_____
_____
_____

What could have made the day better?

_____
_____
_____
_____
_____

How can you better deal with difficulties in the future?

_____
_____
_____
_____
_____

What can you be grateful for today?

_____
_____
_____
_____
_____

Rate the Day

★ ★ ★ ★ ★

Date: ___ / ___ / ___   M T W T F S S

Hours of Sleep: _____

Today's Mood

😄 😊 😐 🙁 😣

Morning: Afternoon: Evening:

_____   _____   _____

_____   _____   _____

_____   _____   _____

Did you feel any of the following today?

☐ Sad

☐ Hopeless

☐ Nervous

☐ Angry / Frustrated

☐ Low Energy / Fatigue

☐ Difficulty Concentrating

☐ Increase or Decrease in Appetite

☐ Other: _____

Food & Beverages

B: _____

L: _____

D: _____

Other: _____

Water

☐ ☐ ☐ ☐ ☐ ☐ ☐ ☐

What impacted your mood today?

_____

_____

_____

_____

_____

_____

Positive things about today:

_____
_____
_____
_____
_____

What could have made the day better?

_____
_____
_____
_____

How can you better deal with difficulties in the future?

_____
_____
_____
_____

What can you be grateful for today?

_____
_____
_____
_____

Rate the Day

★ ★ ★ ★ ★

Date: / / M T W T F S S
Hours of Sleep: _____

Today's Mood

Morning: _____ Afternoon: _____ Evening: _____
_____ _____ _____
_____ _____ _____

Did you feel any of the following today?

- ☐ Sad
- ☐ Hopeless
- ☐ Nervous
- ☐ Angry / Frustrated
- ☐ Low Energy / Fatigue
- ☐ Difficulty Concentrating
- ☐ Increase or Decrease in Appetite
- ☐ Other: _____

Food & Beverages

B: _____

L: _____

D: _____

Other: _____

Water

☐ ☐ ☐ ☐ ☐ ☐ ☐ ☐

What impacted your mood today?
_____
_____
_____
_____
_____
_____

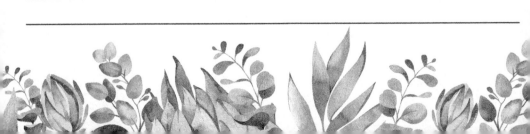

Positive things about today:

_____
_____
_____
_____
_____

What could have made the day better?

_____
_____
_____
_____

How can you better deal with difficulties in the future?

_____
_____
_____
_____

What can you be grateful for today?

_____
_____
_____
_____

Rate the Day

★★★★★

Date: ___ / ___ / ___   M T W T F S S

Hours of Sleep: _____

Today's Mood

Morning: Afternoon: Evening:

_____   _____   _____

_____   _____   _____

_____   _____   _____

Did you feel any of the following today?

☐ Sad

☐ Hopeless

☐ Nervous

☐ Angry / Frustrated

☐ Low Energy / Fatigue

☐ Difficulty Concentrating

☐ Increase or Decrease in Appetite

☐ Other: _____

Food & Beverages

B: _____

L: _____

D: _____

Other: _____

Water

☐ ☐ ☐ ☐ ☐ ☐ ☐ ☐

What impacted your mood today?

_____

_____

_____

_____

_____

_____

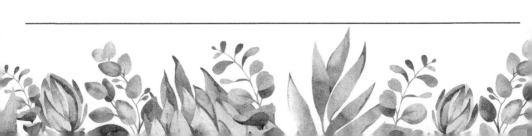

Positive things about today:

_____
_____
_____
_____
_____

What could have made the day better?

_____
_____
_____
_____
_____

How can you better deal with difficulties in the future?

_____
_____
_____
_____
_____

What can you be grateful for today?

_____
_____
_____
_____
_____

Rate the Day

★ ★ ★ ★ ★

Date: ___ / ___ / ___   M T W T F S S

Hours of Sleep: _____

Today's Mood

Morning: _____   Afternoon: _____   Evening: _____

_____   _____   _____

_____   _____   _____

_____   _____   _____

Did you feel any of the following today?

☐ Sad

☐ Hopeless

☐ Nervous

☐ Angry / Frustrated

☐ Low Energy / Fatigue

☐ Difficulty Concentrating

☐ Increase or Decrease in Appetite

☐ Other: _____

Food & Beverages

B: _____

L: _____

D: _____

Other: _____

Water

☐ ☐ ☐ ☐ ☐ ☐ ☐ ☐

What impacted your mood today?

_____

_____

_____

_____

_____

_____

Positive things about today:

_____
_____
_____
_____

What could have made the day better?

_____
_____
_____
_____

How can you better deal with difficulties in the future?

_____
_____
_____
_____

What can you be grateful for today?

_____
_____
_____
_____

Rate the Day

★ ★ ★ ★ ★

Date: /   /   M T W T F S S

Hours of Sleep: _____

Today's Mood

😃 😊 😐 🙁 😢

Morning:
_____
_____
_____

Afternoon:
_____
_____
_____

Evening:
_____
_____
_____

Did you feel any of the following today?

☐ Sad
☐ Hopeless
☐ Nervous
☐ Angry / Frustrated
☐ Low Energy / Fatigue
☐ Difficulty Concentrating
☐ Increase or Decrease in Appetite
☐ Other: _____

Food & Beverages
B: _____
L: _____
D: _____
Other: _____

Water
☐ ☐ ☐ ☐ ☐ ☐ ☐ ☐

What impacted your mood today?
_____
_____
_____
_____
_____
_____

Positive things about today:

_____
_____
_____
_____
_____

What could have made the day better?

_____
_____
_____
_____
_____

How can you better deal with difficulties in the future?

_____
_____
_____
_____
_____

What can you be grateful for today?

_____
_____
_____
_____
_____

Rate the Day

★ ★ ★ ★ ★

Date: / /   M T W T F S S

Hours of Sleep: _____

Today's Mood

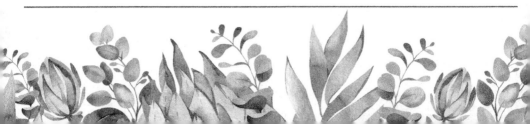

Morning:

_____

_____

_____

Afternoon:

_____

_____

_____

Evening:

_____

_____

_____

Did you feel any of the following today?

- [ ] Sad
- [ ] Hopeless
- [ ] Nervous
- [ ] Angry / Frustrated
- [ ] Low Energy / Fatigue
- [ ] Difficulty Concentrating
- [ ] Increase or Decrease in Appetite
- [ ] Other: _____

Food & Beverages

B: _____

L: _____

D: _____

Other: _____

Water

What impacted your mood today?

_____

_____

_____

_____

_____

_____

Positive things about today:

_____
_____
_____
_____

What could have made the day better?

_____
_____
_____
_____

How can you better deal with difficulties in the future?

_____
_____
_____
_____

What can you be grateful for today?

_____
_____
_____
_____

Rate the Day
★ ★ ★ ★ ★

Date: / / M T W T F S S

Hours of Sleep: _____

Today's Mood

Morning:	Afternoon:	Evening:
_____	_____	_____
_____	_____	_____
_____	_____	_____

Did you feel any of the following today?

☐ Sad
☐ Hopeless
☐ Nervous
☐ Angry / Frustrated
☐ Low Energy / Fatigue
☐ Difficulty Concentrating
☐ Increase or Decrease in Appetite
☐ Other: _____

Food & Beverages

B: _____

L: _____

D: _____

Other: _____

Water

☐ ☐ ☐ ☐ ☐ ☐ ☐ ☐

What impacted your mood today?

_____
_____
_____
_____
_____
_____
_____

Positive things about today:
_____
_____
_____
_____
_____

What could have made the day better?
_____
_____
_____
_____

How can you better deal with difficulties in the future?
_____
_____
_____
_____

What can you be grateful for today?
_____
_____
_____
_____

Rate the Day

★ ★ ★ ★ ★

Date: / /   M T W T F S S

Hours of Sleep: _____

Today's Mood

Morning: _____

Afternoon: _____

Evening: _____

_____

_____

_____

_____

_____

_____

_____

_____

_____

Did you feel any of the following today?

☐ Sad

☐ Hopeless

☐ Nervous

☐ Angry / Frustrated

☐ Low Energy / Fatigue

☐ Difficulty Concentrating

☐ Increase or Decrease in Appetite

☐ Other: _____

Food & Beverages

B: _____

L: _____

D: _____

Other: _____

Water

☐ ☐ ☐ ☐ ☐ ☐ ☐ ☐

What impacted your mood today?

_____

_____

_____

_____

_____

_____

_____

Positive things about today:

_____
_____
_____
_____
_____

What could have made the day better?

_____
_____
_____
_____

How can you better deal with difficulties in the future?

_____
_____
_____
_____

What can you be grateful for today?

_____
_____
_____
_____

Rate the Day

★ ★ ★ ★ ★

Date: / /   M T W T F S S

Hours of Sleep: _____

Today's Mood

Morning: Afternoon: Evening:
_____   _____   _____
_____   _____   _____
_____   _____   _____

Did you feel any of the following
today?

☐ Sad
☐ Hopeless
☐ Nervous
☐ Angry / Frustrated
☐ Low Energy / Fatigue
☐ Difficulty Concentrating
☐ Increase or Decrease in Appetite
☐ Other: _____

Food & Beverages

B: _____

L: _____

D: _____

Other: _____

Water

☐ ☐ ☐ ☐ ☐ ☐ ☐ ☐

What impacted your mood today?
_____
_____
_____
_____
_____
_____

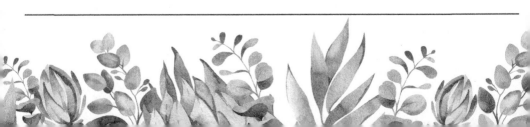

Positive things about today:

_____
_____
_____
_____
_____

What could have made the day better?

_____
_____
_____
_____
_____

How can you better deal with difficulties in the future?

_____
_____
_____
_____
_____

What can you be grateful for today?

_____
_____
_____
_____
_____

Rate the Day

★ ★ ★ ★ ★

Date: / /   M T W T F S S

Hours of Sleep: _____

Today's Mood

Morning: Afternoon: Evening:

_____   _____   _____

_____   _____   _____

_____   _____   _____

Did you feel any of the following today?

☐ Sad

☐ Hopeless

☐ Nervous

☐ Angry / Frustrated

☐ Low Energy / Fatigue

☐ Difficulty Concentrating

☐ Increase or Decrease in Appetite

☐ Other: _____

Food & Beverages

B: _____

L: _____

D: _____

Other: _____

Water

☐ ☐ ☐ ☐ ☐ ☐ ☐ ☐

What impacted your mood today?

_____

_____

_____

_____

_____

_____

Positive things about today:

_____
_____
_____
_____
_____

What could have made the day better?

_____
_____
_____
_____
_____

How can you better deal with difficulties in the future?

_____
_____
_____
_____
_____

What can you be grateful for today?

_____
_____
_____
_____
_____

Rate the Day

★ ★ ★ ★ ★

Date: / /   M T W T F S S

Hours of Sleep: _____

Today's Mood

Morning:

_____

_____

_____

Afternoon:

_____

_____

_____

Evening:

_____

_____

_____

Did you feel any of the following today?

☐ Sad

☐ Hopeless

☐ Nervous

☐ Angry / Frustrated

☐ Low Energy / Fatigue

☐ Difficulty Concentrating

☐ Increase or Decrease in Appetite

☐ Other: _____

Food & Beverages

B: _____

L: _____

D: _____

Other: _____

Water

☐ ☐ ☐ ☐ ☐ ☐ ☐ ☐

What impacted your mood today?

_____

_____

_____

_____

_____

_____

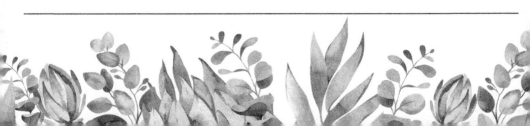

Positive things about today:

_____
_____
_____
_____
_____

What could have made the day better?

_____
_____
_____
_____

How can you better deal with difficulties in the future?

_____
_____
_____
_____

What can you be grateful for today?

_____
_____
_____
_____

Rate the Day

★ ★ ★ ★ ★

Date: / /   M T W T F S S

Hours of Sleep: _____

Today's Mood

Morning: _____   Afternoon: _____   Evening: _____

_____   _____   _____

_____   _____   _____

Did you feel any of the following today?

☐ Sad
☐ Hopeless
☐ Nervous
☐ Angry / Frustrated
☐ Low Energy / Fatigue
☐ Difficulty Concentrating
☐ Increase or Decrease in Appetite
☐ Other: _____

Food & Beverages

B: _____

L: _____

D: _____

Other: _____

Water

☐ ☐ ☐ ☐ ☐ ☐ ☐ ☐

What impacted your mood today?

_____

_____

_____

_____

_____

_____

Positive things about today:

_____
_____
_____
_____

What could have made the day better?

_____
_____
_____
_____

How can you better deal with difficulties in the future?

_____
_____
_____
_____

What can you be grateful for today?

_____
_____
_____
_____

Rate the Day

★★★★★

Date: ___ / ___ / ___   M T W T F S S

Hours of Sleep: _____

Today's Mood

Morning: _____   Afternoon: _____   Evening: _____

_____   _____   _____

_____   _____   _____

_____   _____   _____

Did you feel any of the following today?

- [ ] Sad
- [ ] Hopeless
- [ ] Nervous
- [ ] Angry / Frustrated
- [ ] Low Energy / Fatigue
- [ ] Difficulty Concentrating
- [ ] Increase or Decrease in Appetite
- [ ] Other: _____

Food & Beverages

B: _____

L: _____

D: _____

Other: _____

Water

- [ ] [ ] [ ] [ ] [ ] [ ] [ ] [ ]

What impacted your mood today?

_____

_____

_____

_____

_____

_____

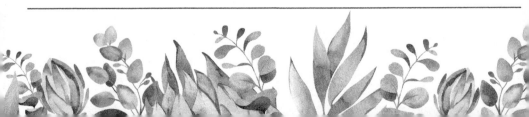

Positive things about today:

_____
_____
_____
_____
_____

What could have made the day better?

_____
_____
_____
_____

How can you better deal with difficulties in the future?

_____
_____
_____
_____

What can you be grateful for today?

_____
_____
_____
_____

Rate the Day

★ ★ ★ ★ ★

Date: /   /   M T W T F S S

Hours of Sleep: _____

Today's Mood

Morning: Afternoon: Evening:

_____   _____   _____

_____   _____   _____

_____   _____   _____

Did you feel any of the following today?

☐ Sad

☐ Hopeless

☐ Nervous

☐ Angry / Frustrated

☐ Low Energy / Fatigue

☐ Difficulty Concentrating

☐ Increase or Decrease in Appetite

☐ Other: _____

Food & Beverages

B: _____

L: _____

D: _____

Other: _____

Water

☐ ☐ ☐ ☐ ☐ ☐ ☐ ☐

What impacted your mood today?

_____

_____

_____

_____

_____

_____

Positive things about today:

_____

_____

_____

_____

What could have made the day better?

_____

_____

_____

_____

How can you better deal with difficulties in the future?

_____

_____

_____

_____

What can you be grateful for today?

_____

_____

_____

_____

Rate the Day

★ ★ ★ ★ ★

Date: ___/___/___ M T W T F S S

Hours of Sleep: _____

Today's Mood

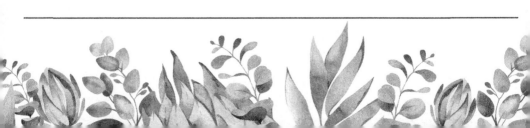

Morning: _____ Afternoon: _____ Evening: _____

_____ _____ _____

_____ _____ _____

_____ _____ _____

Did you feel any of the following today?

☐ Sad

☐ Hopeless

☐ Nervous

☐ Angry / Frustrated

☐ Low Energy / Fatigue

☐ Difficulty Concentrating

☐ Increase or Decrease in Appetite

☐ Other: _____

Food & Beverages

B: _____

L: _____

D: _____

Other: _____

Water

☐ ☐ ☐ ☐ ☐ ☐ ☐ ☐

What impacted your mood today?

_____

_____

_____

_____

_____

_____

Positive things about today:

_____
_____
_____
_____
_____

What could have made the day better?

_____
_____
_____
_____

How can you better deal with difficulties in the future?

_____
_____
_____
_____
_____

What can you be grateful for today?

_____
_____
_____
_____

Rate the Day

★ ★ ★ ★ ★

Date: / /   M T W T F S S
Hours of Sleep: _____

Today's Mood

Morning: Afternoon: Evening:
_____   _____   _____
_____   _____   _____
_____   _____   _____

Did you feel any of the following today?

☐ Sad
☐ Hopeless
☐ Nervous
☐ Angry / Frustrated
☐ Low Energy / Fatigue
☐ Difficulty Concentrating
☐ Increase or Decrease in Appetite
☐ Other: _____

Food & Beverages
B: _____
L: _____
D: _____
Other: _____

Water
☐ ☐ ☐ ☐ ☐ ☐ ☐ ☐

What impacted your mood today?
_____
_____
_____
_____
_____
_____

Positive things about today:

_____
_____
_____
_____
_____

What could have made the day better?

_____
_____
_____
_____

How can you better deal with difficulties in the future?

_____
_____
_____
_____

What can you be grateful for today?

_____
_____
_____
_____

Rate the Day

★ ★ ★ ★ ★

Date: ___ / ___ / ___   M T W T F S S

Hours of Sleep: _____

Today's Mood

Morning: Afternoon: Evening:
_____   _____   _____
_____   _____   _____
_____   _____   _____

Did you feel any of the following today?

☐ Sad
☐ Hopeless
☐ Nervous
☐ Angry / Frustrated
☐ Low Energy / Fatigue
☐ Difficulty Concentrating
☐ Increase or Decrease in Appetite
☐ Other: _____

Food & Beverages
B: _____
L: _____
D: _____
Other: _____

Water
☐ ☐ ☐ ☐ ☐ ☐ ☐ ☐

What impacted your mood today?
_____
_____
_____
_____
_____
_____

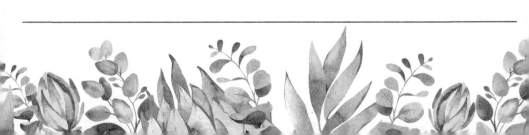

Positive things about today:

_____
_____
_____
_____
_____

What could have made the day better?

_____
_____
_____
_____

How can you better deal with difficulties in the future?

_____
_____
_____
_____

What can you be grateful for today?

_____
_____
_____
_____

Rate the Day

★ ★ ★ ★ ★

Date: / / M T W T F S S

Hours of Sleep: _____

Today's Mood

Morning: _____

Afternoon: _____

Evening: _____

_____ _____ _____

_____ _____ _____

Did you feel any of the following today?

- [ ] Sad
- [ ] Hopeless
- [ ] Nervous
- [ ] Angry / Frustrated
- [ ] Low Energy / Fatigue
- [ ] Difficulty Concentrating
- [ ] Increase or Decrease in Appetite
- [ ] Other: _____

Food & Beverages

B: _____

L: _____

D: _____

Other: _____

Water

- [ ] [ ] [ ] [ ] [ ] [ ] [ ] [ ]

What impacted your mood today?

_____

_____

_____

_____

_____

_____

Positive things about today:

_____
_____
_____
_____
_____

What could have made the day better?

_____
_____
_____
_____

How can you better deal with difficulties in the future?

_____
_____
_____
_____

What can you be grateful for today?

_____
_____
_____
_____

Rate the Day

★ ★ ★ ★ ★

Date: / /   M T W T F S S

Hours of Sleep: _____

Today's Mood

Morning: Afternoon: Evening:

_____   _____   _____

_____   _____   _____

_____   _____   _____

Did you feel any of the following today?

- [ ] Sad
- [ ] Hopeless
- [ ] Nervous
- [ ] Angry / Frustrated
- [ ] Low Energy / Fatigue
- [ ] Difficulty Concentrating
- [ ] Increase or Decrease in Appetite
- [ ] Other: _____

Food & Beverages

B: _____

L: _____

D: _____

Other: _____

Water

- [ ] [ ] [ ] [ ] [ ] [ ] [ ] [ ]

What impacted your mood today?

_____

_____

_____

_____

_____

_____

Positive things about today:

_____
_____
_____
_____
_____

What could have made the day better?

_____
_____
_____
_____

How can you better deal with difficulties in the future?

_____
_____
_____
_____

What can you be grateful for today?

_____
_____
_____
_____

Rate the Day

★ ★ ★ ★ ★

Date: ___/___/___   M T W T F S S

Hours of Sleep: _____

Today's Mood

Morning: _____   Afternoon: _____   Evening: _____

_____   _____   _____

_____   _____   _____

_____   _____   _____

Did you feel any of the following today?

☐ Sad

☐ Hopeless

☐ Nervous

☐ Angry / Frustrated

☐ Low Energy / Fatigue

☐ Difficulty Concentrating

☐ Increase or Decrease in Appetite

☐ Other: _____

Food & Beverages

B: _____

L: _____

D: _____

Other: _____

Water

☐ ☐ ☐ ☐ ☐ ☐ ☐ ☐

What impacted your mood today?

_____

_____

_____

_____

_____

_____

Positive things about today:

_____
_____
_____
_____
_____

What could have made the day better?

_____
_____
_____
_____
_____

How can you better deal with difficulties in the future?

_____
_____
_____
_____
_____

What can you be grateful for today?

_____
_____
_____
_____
_____

Rate the Day

★ ★ ★ ★ ★

Date: / /   M T W T F S S

Hours of Sleep: _____

Today's Mood

Morning: Afternoon: Evening:
_____   _____   _____
_____   _____   _____
_____   _____   _____

Did you feel any of the following today?

☐ Sad
☐ Hopeless
☐ Nervous
☐ Angry / Frustrated
☐ Low Energy / Fatigue
☐ Difficulty Concentrating
☐ Increase or Decrease in Appetite
☐ Other: _____

Food & Beverages

B: _____

L: _____

D: _____

Other: _____

Water

☐ ☐ ☐ ☐ ☐ ☐ ☐ ☐

What impacted your mood today?
_____
_____
_____
_____
_____
_____

Positive things about today:

_____
_____
_____
_____
_____

What could have made the day better?

_____
_____
_____
_____

How can you better deal with difficulties in the future?

_____
_____
_____
_____

What can you be grateful for today?

_____
_____
_____
_____

Rate the Day

★ ★ ★ ★ ★

Date: ___/___/___ M T W T F S S

Hours of Sleep: _____

Today's Mood

😃 🙂 😐 🙁 😢

Morning: Afternoon: Evening:

_____   _____   _____

_____   _____   _____

_____   _____   _____

Did you feel any of the following today?

☐ Sad

☐ Hopeless

☐ Nervous

☐ Angry / Frustrated

☐ Low Energy / Fatigue

☐ Difficulty Concentrating

☐ Increase or Decrease in Appetite

☐ Other: _____

Food & Beverages

B: _____

L: _____

D: _____

Other: _____

Water

🥛 🥛 🥛 🥛 🥛 🥛 🥛 🥛

☐ ☐ ☐ ☐ ☐ ☐ ☐ ☐

What impacted your mood today?

_____

_____

_____

_____

_____

_____

Positive things about today:

_____
_____
_____
_____
_____

What could have made the day better?

_____
_____
_____
_____

How can you better deal with difficulties in the future?

_____
_____
_____
_____

What can you be grateful for today?

_____
_____
_____
_____

Rate the Day

★ ★ ★ ★ ★

Date: /   /   M T W T F S S

Hours of Sleep: _____

Today's Mood

Morning: Afternoon: Evening:
_____   _____   _____
_____   _____   _____
_____   _____   _____

Did you feel any of the following today?

☐ Sad
☐ Hopeless
☐ Nervous
☐ Angry / Frustrated
☐ Low Energy / Fatigue
☐ Difficulty Concentrating
☐ Increase or Decrease in Appetite
☐ Other: _____

Food & Beverages

B: _____
L: _____
D: _____
Other: _____

Water

☐ ☐ ☐ ☐ ☐ ☐ ☐ ☐

What impacted your mood today?
_____
_____
_____
_____
_____
_____

Positive things about today:

_____
_____
_____
_____
_____

What could have made the day better?

_____
_____
_____
_____

How can you better deal with difficulties in the future?

_____
_____
_____
_____

What can you be grateful for today?

_____
_____
_____
_____

Rate the Day

★ ★ ★ ★ ★

Date: / / M T W T F S S

Hours of Sleep: _____

Today's Mood

Morning: _____ Afternoon: _____ Evening: _____
_____ _____ _____
_____ _____ _____

Did you feel any of the following today?

☐ Sad
☐ Hopeless
☐ Nervous
☐ Angry / Frustrated
☐ Low Energy / Fatigue
☐ Difficulty Concentrating
☐ Increase or Decrease in Appetite
☐ Other: _____

Food & Beverages

B: _____
L: _____
D: _____
Other: _____

Water

☐ ☐ ☐ ☐ ☐ ☐ ☐ ☐

What impacted your mood today?
_____
_____
_____
_____
_____
_____

Positive things about today:

_____

_____

_____

_____

_____

What could have made the day better?

_____

_____

_____

_____

_____

How can you better deal with difficulties in the future?

_____

_____

_____

_____

_____

What can you be grateful for today?

_____

_____

_____

_____

_____

Rate the Day

★ ★ ★ ★ ★

Date: / / M T W T F S S

Hours of Sleep: _____

Today's Mood

Morning: _____ Afternoon: _____ Evening: _____

_____ _____ _____

_____ _____ _____

Did you feel any of the following today?

☐ Sad

☐ Hopeless

☐ Nervous

☐ Angry / Frustrated

☐ Low Energy / Fatigue

☐ Difficulty Concentrating

☐ Increase or Decrease in Appetite

☐ Other: _____

Food & Beverages

B: _____

L: _____

D: _____

Other:

Water

☐ ☐ ☐ ☐ ☐ ☐ ☐ ☐

What impacted your mood today?

_____

_____

_____

_____

_____

_____

Positive things about today:

_____
_____
_____
_____
_____

What could have made the day better?

_____
_____
_____
_____

How can you better deal with difficulties in the future?

_____
_____
_____
_____

What can you be grateful for today?

_____
_____
_____
_____

Rate the Day

★ ★ ★ ★ ★

Date: ___ / ___ / ___   M T W T F S S

Hours of Sleep: _____

Today's Mood

😄 😊 😐 🙁 😢

Morning: Afternoon: Evening:

_____   _____   _____

_____   _____   _____

_____   _____   _____

Did you feel any of the following today?

☐ Sad

☐ Hopeless

☐ Nervous

☐ Angry / Frustrated

☐ Low Energy / Fatigue

☐ Difficulty Concentrating

☐ Increase or Decrease in Appetite

☐ Other: _____

Food & Beverages

B: _____

L: _____

D: _____

Other: _____

Water

☐ ☐ ☐ ☐ ☐ ☐ ☐ ☐

What impacted your mood today?

_____

_____

_____

_____

_____

_____

Positive things about today:

_____
_____
_____
_____
_____

What could have made the day better?

_____
_____
_____
_____

How can you better deal with difficulties in the future?

_____
_____
_____
_____

What can you be grateful for today?

_____
_____
_____
_____

Rate the Day

★ ★ ★ ★ ★

Date: /   /   M T W T F S S

Hours of Sleep: _____

Today's Mood

Morning: Afternoon: Evening:

_____   _____   _____

_____   _____   _____

_____   _____   _____

Did you feel any of the following today?

- [ ] Sad
- [ ] Hopeless
- [ ] Nervous
- [ ] Angry / Frustrated
- [ ] Low Energy / Fatigue
- [ ] Difficulty Concentrating
- [ ] Increase or Decrease in Appetite
- [ ] Other: _____

Food & Beverages

B: _____

L: _____

D: _____

Other: _____

Water

☐ ☐ ☐ ☐ ☐ ☐ ☐ ☐

What impacted your mood today?

_____

_____

_____

_____

_____

Positive things about today:

_____
_____
_____
_____
_____

What could have made the day better?

_____
_____
_____
_____
_____

How can you better deal with difficulties in the future?

_____
_____
_____
_____
_____

What can you be grateful for today?

_____
_____
_____
_____
_____

Rate the Day

⭐ ⭐ ⭐ ⭐ ⭐

Date: ___ / ___ / ___   M T W T F S S

Hours of Sleep: _____

Today's Mood

😄 😊 😐 🙁 😢

Morning: | Afternoon: | Evening:
_____ | _____ | _____
_____ | _____ | _____
_____ | _____ | _____

Did you feel any of the following today?

☐ Sad

☐ Hopeless

☐ Nervous

☐ Angry / Frustrated

☐ Low Energy / Fatigue

☐ Difficulty Concentrating

☐ Increase or Decrease in Appetite

☐ Other: _____

Food & Beverages

B: _____

L: _____

D: _____

Other: _____

Water

☐ ☐ ☐ ☐ ☐ ☐ ☐ ☐

What impacted your mood today?

_____

_____

_____

_____

_____

_____

Positive things about today:

_____
_____
_____
_____
_____

What could have made the day better?

_____
_____
_____
_____

How can you better deal with difficulties in the future?

_____
_____
_____
_____

What can you be grateful for today?

_____
_____
_____
_____

Rate the Day

★ ★ ★ ★ ★

Date: / /   M T W T F S S

Hours of Sleep: _____

Today's Mood

Morning: Afternoon: Evening:
_____   _____   _____
_____   _____   _____
_____   _____   _____

Did you feel any of the following today?

- [ ] Sad
- [ ] Hopeless
- [ ] Nervous
- [ ] Angry / Frustrated
- [ ] Low Energy / Fatigue
- [ ] Difficulty Concentrating
- [ ] Increase or Decrease in Appetite
- [ ] Other: _____

Food & Beverages

B: _____

L: _____

D: _____

Other: _____

Water

- [ ] [ ] [ ] [ ] [ ] [ ] [ ] [ ]

What impacted your mood today?
_____
_____
_____
_____
_____
_____

Positive things about today:

_____
_____
_____
_____
_____

What could have made the day better?

_____
_____
_____
_____

How can you better deal with difficulties in the future?

_____
_____
_____
_____

What can you be grateful for today?

_____
_____
_____
_____

Rate the Day

★ ★ ★ ★ ★

Date: / / M T W T F S S

Hours of Sleep: _____

Today's Mood

Morning: | Afternoon: | Evening:
_____

_____

_____

Did you feel any of the following today?

- [ ] Sad
- [ ] Hopeless
- [ ] Nervous
- [ ] Angry / Frustrated
- [ ] Low Energy / Fatigue
- [ ] Difficulty Concentrating
- [ ] Increase or Decrease in Appetite
- [ ] Other: _____

Food & Beverages

B: _____

L: _____

D: _____

Other: _____

Water

What impacted your mood today?

_____

_____

_____

_____

_____

Positive things about today:

_____
_____
_____
_____

What could have made the day better?

_____
_____
_____
_____

How can you better deal with difficulties in the future?

_____
_____
_____
_____

What can you be grateful for today?

_____
_____
_____
_____

Rate the Day

★ ★ ★ ★ ★

Date: ___ / ___ / ___   M T W T F S S

Hours of Sleep: _____

Today's Mood

😁 😊 😐 🙁 😣

Morning: **Afternoon:**   **Evening:**

_____   _____   _____

_____   _____   _____

_____   _____   _____

Did you feel any of the following today?

☐ Sad

☐ Hopeless

☐ Nervous

☐ Angry / Frustrated

☐ Low Energy / Fatigue

☐ Difficulty Concentrating

☐ Increase or Decrease in Appetite

☐ Other: _____

Food & Beverages
B: _____
L: _____
D: _____
Other: _____

Water

🥛 🥛 🥛 🥛 🥛 🥛 🥛 🥛

☐ ☐ ☐ ☐ ☐ ☐ ☐ ☐

What impacted your mood today?

_____

_____

_____

_____

_____

_____

Positive things about today:

_____
_____
_____
_____
_____

What could have made the day better?

_____
_____
_____
_____

How can you better deal with difficulties in the future?

_____
_____
_____
_____

What can you be grateful for today?

_____
_____
_____
_____

Rate the Day

★ ★ ★ ★ ★

Date: ___ / ___ / ___ M T W T F S S

Hours of Sleep: _____

Today's Mood

Morning: | Afternoon: | Evening:

_____ _____ _____
_____ _____ _____
_____ _____ _____

Did you feel any of the following today?

☐ Sad

☐ Hopeless

☐ Nervous

☐ Angry / Frustrated

☐ Low Energy / Fatigue

☐ Difficulty Concentrating

☐ Increase or Decrease in Appetite

☐ Other: _____

Food & Beverages

B: _____

L: _____

D: _____

Other: _____

Water

☐ ☐ ☐ ☐ ☐ ☐ ☐ ☐

What impacted your mood today?

_____

_____

_____

_____

_____

_____

Positive things about today:

_____
_____
_____
_____
_____

What could have made the day better?

_____
_____
_____
_____

How can you better deal with difficulties in the future?

_____
_____
_____
_____

What can you be grateful for today?

_____
_____
_____
_____

Rate the Day

★ ★ ★ ★ ★

Date: /   /   M   T   W   T   F   S   S

Hours of Sleep: _____

Today's Mood

Morning: Afternoon: Evening:

_____   _____   _____

_____   _____   _____

_____   _____   _____

Did you feel any of the following today?

☐ Sad

☐ Hopeless

☐ Nervous

☐ Angry / Frustrated

☐ Low Energy / Fatigue

☐ Difficulty Concentrating

☐ Increase or Decrease in Appetite

☐ Other: _____

Food & Beverages

B: _____

L: _____

D: _____

Other: _____

Water

☐ ☐ ☐ ☐ ☐ ☐ ☐ ☐

What impacted your mood today?

_____

_____

_____

_____

_____

_____

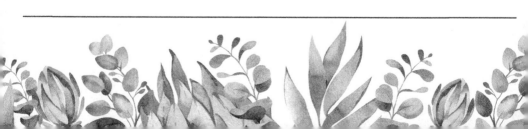

Positive things about today:

_____
_____
_____
_____
_____

What could have made the day better?

_____
_____
_____
_____
_____

How can you better deal with difficulties in the future?

_____
_____
_____
_____
_____

What can you be grateful for today?

_____
_____
_____
_____
_____

Rate the Day

★ ★ ★ ★ ★

Date: /   /   M T W T F S S
Hours of Sleep: _____

Today's Mood

Morning: Afternoon: Evening:
_____   _____   _____
_____   _____   _____
_____   _____   _____

Did you feel any of the following today?

☐ Sad
☐ Hopeless
☐ Nervous
☐ Angry / Frustrated
☐ Low Energy / Fatigue
☐ Difficulty Concentrating
☐ Increase or Decrease in Appetite
☐ Other: _____

Food & Beverages

B: _____
L: _____
D: _____
Other: _____

Water

☐ ☐ ☐ ☐ ☐ ☐ ☐ ☐

What impacted your mood today?
_____
_____
_____
_____
_____
_____

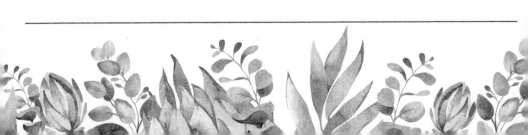

Positive things about today:

_____
_____
_____
_____
_____

What could have made the day better?

_____
_____
_____
_____

How can you better deal with difficulties in the future?

_____
_____
_____
_____

What can you be grateful for today?

_____
_____
_____
_____

Rate the Day

★ ★ ★ ★ ★

Date: / /   M T W T F S S
Hours of Sleep: _____

Today's Mood

Morning: | Afternoon: | Evening:
_____ | _____ | _____
_____ | _____ | _____
_____ | _____ | _____

Did you feel any of the following today?

- [ ] Sad
- [ ] Hopeless
- [ ] Nervous
- [ ] Angry / Frustrated
- [ ] Low Energy / Fatigue
- [ ] Difficulty Concentrating
- [ ] Increase or Decrease in Appetite
- [ ] Other: _____

Food & Beverages

B: _____

L: _____

D: _____

Other: _____

Water

- [ ] [ ] [ ] [ ] [ ] [ ] [ ] [ ]

What impacted your mood today?
_____
_____
_____
_____
_____
_____

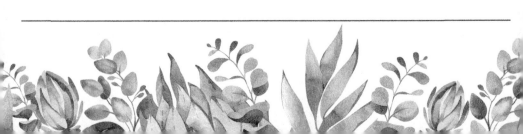

Positive things about today:

_____
_____
_____
_____
_____

What could have made the day better?

_____
_____
_____
_____
_____

How can you better deal with difficulties in the future?

_____
_____
_____
_____
_____

What can you be grateful for today?

_____
_____
_____
_____
_____

Rate the Day

★★★★★